The Definitive Mediterranean Breakfast Guide for Busy People

Easy and Affordable Recipes to Stay Healthy and Start Your Day with a Smile

Ava Foster

Table of contents

Pasta with Pesto

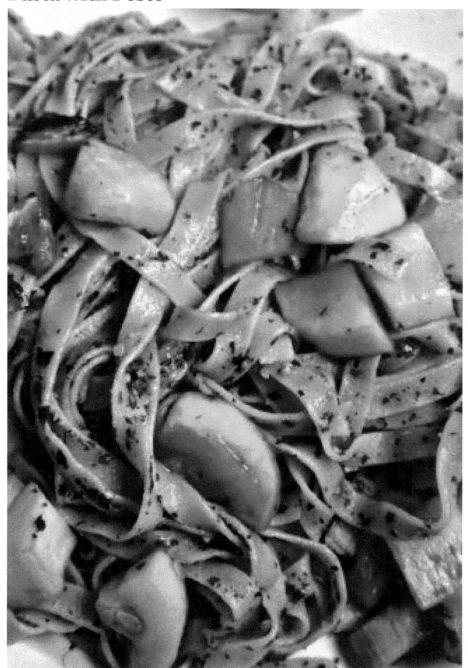

Difficulty Level: 2/5

Preparation time: 10 minutes

Cooking time: 0 minutes

Servings: 4

Ingredients:

3 tablespoons extra-virgin olive oil

3 garlic cloves, finely minced

½ cup fresh basil leaves

¼ cup (about 2 ounces) grated Parmesan cheese

¼ cup pine nuts

8 ounces whole-wheat pasta, cooked according to package instructions and drained

Directions:

In a blender or food processor, combine the olive oil, garlic, basil, cheese, and pine nuts. Pulse for 10 to 20 (1-second) pulses until everything is chopped and blended.

Toss with the hot pasta and serve.

Nutrition:
Calories: 405;

Protein: 13g;

Total Carbohydrates: 44g;

Sugars: 2g;

Fiber: 5g;

Total Fat: 21g;

Saturated Fat: 4g;

Cholesterol: 10mg;

Sodium: 141mg

Breakfast Egg on Avocado

Difficulty Level: 2/5

Preparation time: 10 minutes

Cooking Time: 15 minutes

Servings: 6

Ingredients:

1 tsp garlic powder

1/2 tsp sea salt

1/4 cup Parmesan cheese (grated or shredded)

1/4 tsp black pepper

3 medium avocados (cut in half, pitted, skin on)

6 medium eggs

Directions:

Prepare muffin tins and preheat the oven to 350° F.

To ensure that the egg would fit inside the cavity of the avocado, lightly scrape off 1/3 of the meat.

Place avocado on muffin tin to ensure that it faces with the top up.

Evenly season each avocado with pepper, salt, and garlic powder.

Add one egg on each avocado cavity and garnish tops with cheese.

Pop in the oven and bake until the egg white is set, about 15 minutes.

Serve and enjoy.

Nutrition:

Calories 252;

Protein 14 g;

Carbohydrates 4 g;

Fat 20 g

Egg Muffins with Vegetables and Feta Cheese

Difficulty Level: 2/5

Preparation time: 10 minutes

Cooking time: 15 minutes

Servings: 6

Ingredients:

1 cup finely chopped baby spinach

½ cup chopped tomatoes

½ tablespoon chopped fresh oregano

4 eggs, well beaten

½ cup crumbled feta cheese

¼ cup finely chopped onions

¼ cup chopped, pitted Kalamata olives

1 teaspoon sunflower oil + extra to grease

½ cup cooked quinoa

Directions:

Grease a 6 counts muffin tin with some oil.

Heat a skillet over medium flame and add oil. Add onions and cook until they turn translucent.

Stir in the tomatoes and cook for a minute. Stir in the spinach and cook until it wilts.

Remove from heat.

Add olives and oregano and mix well.

Add quinoa, salt, and feta cheese into the bowl of beaten eggs and whisk well.

Add the sautéed vegetables and mix well.

Spoon into prepared muffin tins.

Bake in a preheated oven at 350° F for about 25 – 30 minutes or until it is done and the top is light golden brown.

Remove from the oven and cool for a few minutes.

Run a knife around the edges of the muffin and loosen the muffins. Invert onto a plate and serve.

Nutrition:

Calories 114;

Fat 7 g;

Carbohydrates 6 g;

Fiber 1 g;

Protein 7 g

Mediterranean Breakfast Stir Fry (Melamen)

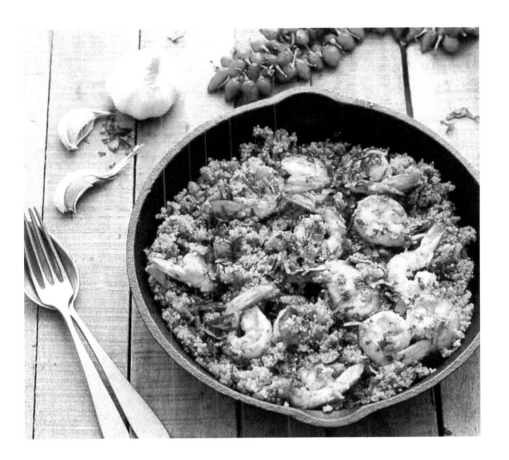

Difficulty Level: 2/5

Preparation time: 10 minutes

Cooking time: 15 minutes

Servings: 8

Ingredients:

3 cups chopped onions

3 cups green bell peppers, chopped

4 large tomatoes, chopped

2 tablespoons extra-virgin olive oil

2 eggs, beaten

Pepper to taste

Salt to taste

Directions:

Heat a pan over a high flame. Add oil and then add bell pepper and sauté for a couple of minutes.

Reduce heat, cover and cook for two minutes.

Add onions and stir. Cover and cook for four to five minutes.

Add tomatoes, salt and pepper, stir and cover again. Cook until the tomatoes are soft.

Pour the beaten egg over the veggies in the pan. Do not stir at all. Let it simmer for 50 to 60 seconds.

Serve with pita bread, cucumbers, and low fat feta cheese.

Nutrition:

Calories 108.7;

Fat 5.1 g;

Carbohydrates 14.3 g;

Fiber 3 g;

Protein 3.6 g

Paleo Almond Banana Pancakes

Difficulty Level: 2/5

Preparation time: 10 minutes

Cooking Time: 10 minutes

Servings: 3

Ingredients:

¼ cup almond flour

½ teaspoon ground cinnamon

3 eggs

1 banana, mashed

1 tablespoon almond butter

1 teaspoon vanilla extract

1 teaspoon olive oil

Sliced banana to serve

Directions:

Whisk the eggs in a mixing bowl until they become fluffy.

In another bowl, mash the banana using a fork and add to the egg mixture.

Add the vanilla, almond butter, cinnamon and almond flour.

Mix into a smooth batter.

Heat the olive oil in a skillet.

Add one spoonful of the batter and fry them on both sides.

Keep doing these steps until you are done with all the batter.

Add some sliced banana on top before serving.

Nutrition:

Calories 306;

Protein 14.4 g;

Carbohydrates 3.6 g;

Fat 26 g

Spinach and Artichoke Frittata

Difficulty Level: 2/5

Preparation time: 5 minutes

Cooking time: 22 minutes to 25 minutes

Servings: 4 to 6

Ingredients:

10 Big eggs

½ cup Full-fat acrid cream

1 tablespoon Dijon mustard

1 teaspoon Genuine salt

¼ teaspoon Crisply ground dark pepper

1 cup Ground parmesan cheddar (around 3 ounces), divided

2 tablespoons

Olive oil

About 14 ounces

Marinated artichoke hearts, depleted, tapped dry, and quartered

5 ounces Infant spinach (around 5 pressed cups)

2 cloves

Garlic, minced

Directions:

Arrange a rack in the broiler and heat to 400° F.

Place the eggs, harsh cream, mustard, salt, pepper and ½ cup of the parmesan in a huge bowl and race to consolidate; put in a safe place.

Heat the oil in a 10 inch cast iron or broiler safe nonstick skillet over medium heat until gleaming. Include the artichokes in a solitary layer and cook, blending occasionally, until delicately caramelized, 6 to 8 minutes. Include the spinach and garlic, and hurl until the spinach is withered and practically all of the fluid is vanished, around 2 minutes.

Spread everything into an even layer. Pour the egg blend over the vegetables. Sprinkle with the staying ½ cup parmesan. Tilt the skillet to ensure the eggs settle uniformly over all the vegetables. Cook undisturbed until the eggs at the edges of the skillet start to set, 2 to 3 minutes.

Bake until the eggs are totally set, 12 to 15 minutes. To check, cut a small cut in the focal point of the frittata. If crude eggs run into the cut, heat for an additional couple of moments. Cool in the search for gold minutes, at that point cut into wedges and serve warm.

Nutritional values based on 6 serving (% day by day esteem):

Calories 316;

Fat 25.9 g (39.9%);

Saturated 7.8 g (38.9%);

Carbs 6.4 g (2.1%);

Fiber 2.3 g (9.3%);

Sugars 2.1 g;

Protein 17.9 g (35.7%);

Sodium 565.2 mg (23.6%)

Banana-Coconut Breakfast

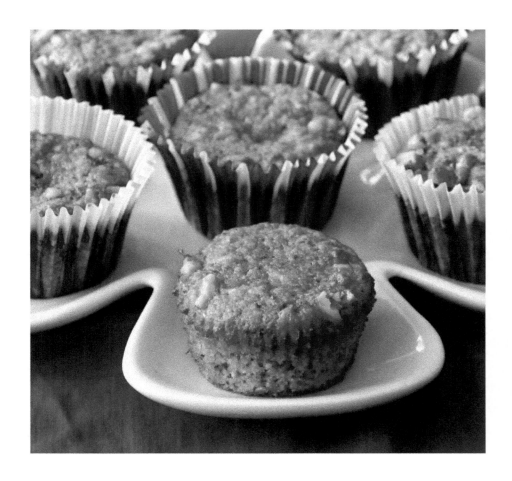

Difficulty Level: 2/5

Preparation time: 10 minutes

Cooking Time: 3 minutes

Servings: 4

Ingredients:

1 ripe banana

1 cup desiccated coconut

1 cup coconut milk

3 tablespoons raisins, chopped

2 tablespoon ground flax seed

1 teaspoon vanilla

A dash of cinnamon

A dash of nutmeg

Salt to taste

Directions:

Place all ingredients in a deep pan.

Allow to simmer for 3 minutes on low heat.

Place in individual containers.

Put a label and store in the fridge.

Allow to thaw at room temperature before heating in the microwave oven.

Nutrition:

Calories per serving 279;

Carbohydrates 25.46 g;

Protein 6.4 g;

Fat 8.8 g;

Fiber 5.9g

Portobello Mushroom Pizza

Difficulty Level: 2/5

Preparation time: 10 minutes

Cooking Time: 12 minutes

Servings: 4

Ingredients:

½ teaspoon red pepper flakes

A handful of fresh basil, chopped

1 can black olives, chopped

1 medium onion, chopped

1 green pepper, chopped

¼ cup chopped roasted yellow peppers

½ cup prepared nut cheese, shredded

2 cups prepared gluten-free pizza sauce

8 Portobello mushrooms, cleaned and stems removed

Directions:

Preheat the oven toaster.

Take a baking sheet and grease it. Set aside.

Place the Portobello mushroom cap-side down and spoon 2 tablespoon of packaged pizza sauce on the underside of each cap. Add nut cheese and top with the remaining ingredients.

Broil for 12 minutes or until the toppings are wilted.

Nutrition:

Calories 578;

Carbohydrates 73 g;

Protein 24.4 g;

Fat 22.4 g

Amazingly Good Parsley Tabbouleh

Difficulty Level: 2/5

Preparation time: 10 minutes

Cooking Time: 15 minutes

Servings: 4

Ingredients:

¼ cup chopped fresh mint

¼ cup lemon juice

¼ tsp salt

½ cup bulgur

½ tsp minced garlic

1 cup water

1 small cucumber, peeled, seeded and diced

2 cups finely chopped flat-leaf parsley

2 tbsp extra virgin olive oil

2 tomatoes, diced

4 scallions, thinly sliced

Pepper to taste

Directions:

Cook bulgur according to package instructions. Drain and set aside to cool for at least 15 minutes.

In a small bowl, mix pepper, salt, garlic, oil, and lemon juice.

Transfer bulgur into a large salad bowl and mix in scallions, cucumber, tomatoes, mint, and parsley.

Pour in dressing and toss well to coat.

Place bowl in ref until chilled before serving.

Nutrition:

Calories 134.8;

Carbohydrates 13 g;

Protein 7.2 g;

Fat 6 g

Artichokes, Olives & Tuna Pasta

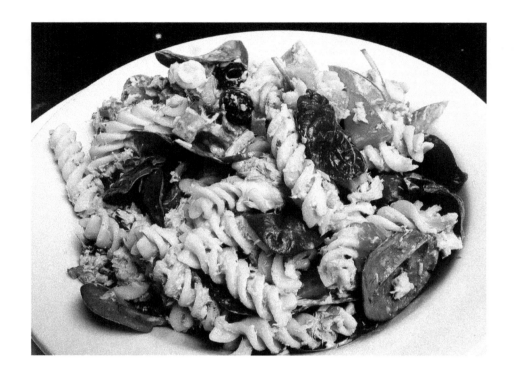

Difficulty Level: 2/5

Preparation time: 10 minutes

Cooking Time: 15 minutes

Servings: 4

Ingredients:

¼ cup chopped fresh basil

¼ cup chopped green olives

¼ tsp freshly ground pepper

½ cup white wine

½ tsp salt, divided

1 10 oz package frozen artichoke hearts, thawed and squeezed dry

2 cups grape tomatoes, halved

2 tbsp lemon juice

2 tsp chopped fresh rosemary

2 tsp freshly grated lemon zest

3 cloves garlic, minced

4 tbsp extra virgin olive oil, divided

6 oz whole wheat penne pasta

8 oz tuna steak, cut into 3 pieces

Directions:

Cook penne pasta according to package instructions. Drain and set aside.

Preheat grill to medium high.

In bowl, toss and mix ¼ tsp pepper, ¼ tsp salt, 1 tsp rosemary, lemon zest, 1 tbsp oil and tuna pieces.

Grill tuna for 3 minutes per side. Allow to cool and flake into bite sized pieces.

On medium fire, place a large nonstick saucepan and heat 3 tbsp oil.

Sauté remaining rosemary, garlic olives, and artichoke hearts for 4 minutes Add wine and tomatoes, bring to a boil and cook for 3 minutes while stirring once in a while.

Add remaining salt, lemon juice, tuna pieces and pasta. Cook until heated through.

To serve, garnish with basil and enjoy.

Nutrition:

Calories 127.6;

Carbohydrates 13 g;

Protein 7.2 g;

Fat 5.2 g

Pork Chops and Tomato Sauce

Difficulty Level: 2/5

Preparation Time: 10 minutes

Cooking Time: 20 minutes

Servings: 4

Ingredients:

4 pork chops, boneless

1 tablespoon soy sauce

¼ teaspoon sesame oil

1 and ½ cups tomato paste

1 yellow onion

8 mushrooms, sliced

Directions:

In a bowl, mix pork chops with soy sauce and sesame oil, toss and leave aside for 10 minutes.

Set your Pressure Pot on sauté mode, add pork chops and brown them for 5 minutes on each side.

Add onion, stir and cook for 1-2 minutes more.

Add tomato paste and mushrooms, toss, cover and cook on high for 8-9 minutes.

Divide everything between plates and serve.

Enjoy!

Nutrition:

Calories 300;

Protein 4 g;

Fat 7 g;

Carbohydrates 18 g

Lamb Coconut Curry

Difficulty Level: 2/5

Preparation Time: 5-8 minutes

Cooking Time: 15 minutes

Servings: 4-5

Ingredients:

2 pounds lamb, diced

A small bunch of lemongrass stalks, trimmed and diced

4 tablespoons minced chili

1 inch pieces ginger root, chopped

1 cup of coconut milk

Directions:

Blend the lemongrass, ginger, and chili in a blender to make a paste.

Place your Pressure Pot over a dry kitchen platform. Open the top lid and plug it on.

Add the paste, lamb, and coconut milk; gently stir to mix well.

Properly close the top lid; make sure that the safety valve is properly locked.

Press "MEAT/STEW" Cooking function; set pressure level to "HIGH" and set the Cooking time to 15 minutes.

Allow the pressure to build to cook the ingredients.

After Cooking time is over press "CANCEL" setting. Find and press "QPR" Cooking function. This setting is for quick release of inside pressure.

Slowly open the lid, take out the cooked recipe in serving containers. Serve warm.

Nutrition:

Calories 524;

Protein 31 g;

Fat 19 g;

Carbohydrates 28g

Crispy Black-Eyed Peas

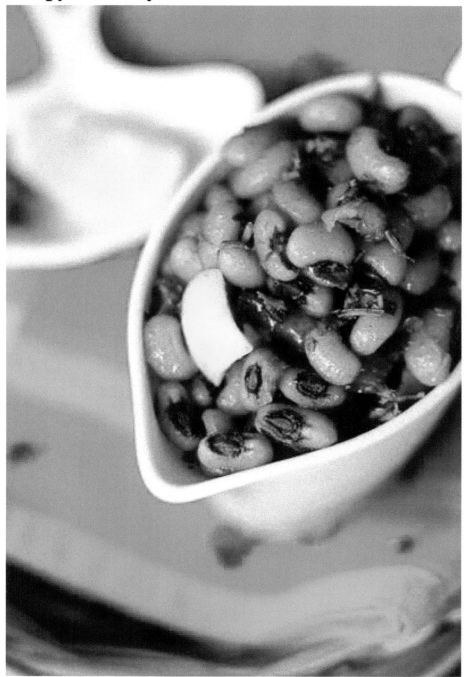

Difficulty Level: 2/5

Preparation Time: 10 minutes

Cooking Time: 15 minutes

Servings: 6

Ingredients:

15 ounces black-eyed peas

1/8 teaspoon chipotle chili powder

¼ teaspoon salt

½ teaspoon chili powder

1/8 teaspoon black pepper

Directions:

Rinse the beans well with running water then set aside. In a large bowl, mix the spices until well combined. Add the peas to spices and mix. Place the peas in the wire basket and cook for

10 minutes at 360° F. Serve and enjoy!

Nutrition:

Calories 262;

Total Fat 9.4 g;

Carbohydrates 8.6 g;

Protein 9.2 g

Spinach Samosa

Difficulty Level: 2/5

Preparation Time: 15 minutes

Cooking Time: 15 minutes

Servings: 2

Ingredients:

1 ½ cups of almond flour

½ teaspoon baking soda

1 teaspoon garam masala

1 teaspoon coriander, chopped

¼ cup green peas

½ teaspoon sesame seeds

¼ cup potatoes, boiled, small chunks

2 tablespoons olive oil

¾ cup boiled and blended spinach puree

Salt and chili powder to taste

Directions:

In a bowl, mix baking soda, salt, and flour to make the dough. Add 1 tablespoon of oil. Add the spinach puree and mix until the dough is smooth.

Place in fridge for 20 minutes.

In the pan add one tablespoon of oil, then add potatoes, peas and cook for 5 minutes.

Add the sesame seeds, garam masala, coriander, and stir.

Knead the dough and make the small ball using a rolling pin. Form balls, make into cone shapes, which are then filled with stuffing that is not yet fully cooked. Make sure flour sheets are well sealed.

Preheat air fryer to 390° F.

Place samosa in air fryer basket and cook for 10 minutes.

Nutrition:

Calories 254;

Total Fat 12.2 g;

Carbohydrates 9.3 g;

Protein 10.2 g

Avocado Fries

Difficulty Level: 2/5

Preparation Time: 10 minutes

Cooking Time: 15 minutes

Servings: 4

Ingredients:

1 ounce Aquafina

1 avocado, sliced

½ teaspoon salt

½ cup panko breadcrumbs

Directions:

Toss the panko breadcrumbs and salt together in a bowl.

Pour Aquafina into another bowl.

Dredge the avocado slices in Aquafina and then panko breadcrumbs.

Arrange the slices in single layer in air fryer basket. Air fry at 390° F for 10 minutes.

Nutrition:

Calories 263;

Total Fat 7.4 g;

Carbohydrates 6.5 g;

Protein 8.2 g

Honey Roasted Carrots

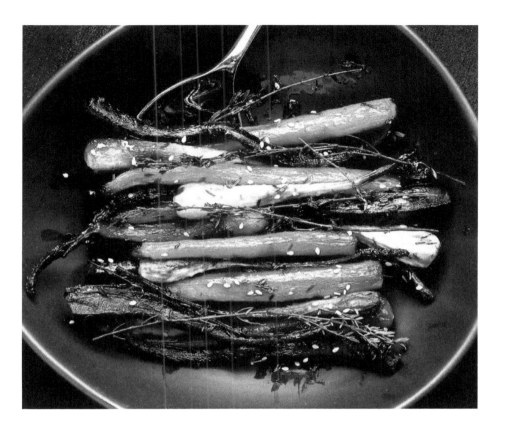

Difficulty Level: 2/5

Preparation Time: 12 minutes

Cooking Time: 15 minutes

Servings: 2

Ingredients:

1 tablespoon honey

Salt and pepper to taste

3 cups of baby carrots

1 tablespoon olive oil

Directions:

In a mixing bowl, combine carrots, honey, and olive oil.

Season with salt and pepper.

Cook in air fryer at 390° F for 12 minutes.

Nutrition:

Calories 257;

Total Fat 11.6 g;

Carbohydrates 8.7 g;

Protein 7.3 g

Full Eggs in a Squash

Difficulty Level: 2/5

Preparation time: 10 minutes

Cooking time: 20 minutes

Servings: 5

Ingredients:

2 acorn squash

6 whole eggs

2 tablespoons extra virgin olive oil

Salt and pepper as needed

5-6 pitted dates

8 walnut halves

A fresh bunch of parsley

Directions:

Pre-heat your oven to 375 degrees Fahrenheit.

Slice squash crosswise and prepare 3 slices with holes.

While slicing the squash, make sure that each slice has a measurement of ¾ inch thickness.

Remove the seeds from the slices.

Take a baking sheet and line it with parchment paper.

Transfer the slices to your baking sheet and season them with salt and pepper.

Bake in your oven for 20 minutes.

Chop the walnuts and dates on your cutting board .

Take the baking dish out of the oven and drizzle slices with olive oil.

Crack an egg into each of the holes in the slices and season with pepper and salt.

Sprinkle the chopped walnuts on top.

Bake for 10 minutes more.

Garnish with parsley and add maple syrup.

Enjoy!

Nutrition (Per Serving)

Calories: 198

Fat: 12g

Carbohydrates: 17g

Protein: 8g

The Great Barley Porridge

Difficulty Level: 2/5

Preparation time: 5 minutes

Cooking time: 25 minutes

Servings: 4

Ingredients:

1 cup barley

1 cup wheat berries

2 cups unsweetened almond milk

2 cups water

½ cup blueberries

½ cup pomegranate seeds

½ cup hazelnuts, toasted and chopped

¼ cup honey

Directions:

Take a medium saucepan and place it over medium-high heat.

Place barley, almond milk, wheat berries, water and bring to a boil.

Reduce the heat to low and simmer for 25 minutes.

Divide amongst serving bowls and top each serving with 2 tablespoons blueberries, 2 tablespoons pomegranate seeds, 2 tablespoons hazelnuts, 1 tablespoon honey.

Serve and enjoy!

Nutrition (Per Serving)

Calories: 295

Fat: 8g

Carbohydrates: 56g

Protein: 6g

Tomato and Dill Frittata

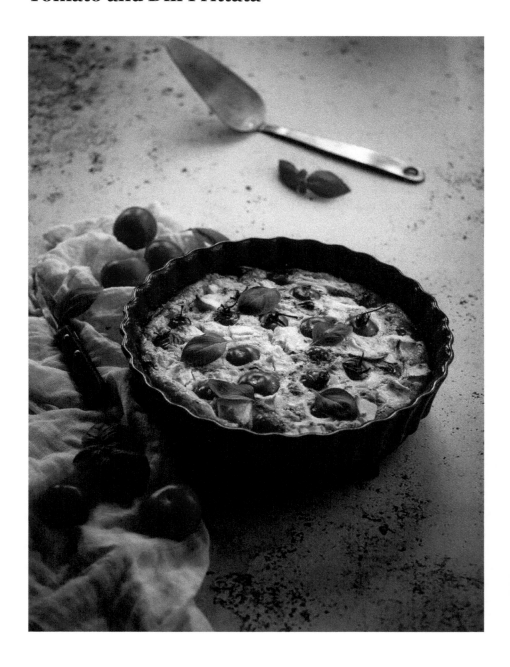

Difficulty Level: 2/5

Preparation time: 5 minutes

Cooking time: 10 minutes

Servings: 4

Ingredients:

2 tablespoons olive oil

1 medium onion, chopped

1 teaspoon garlic, minced

2 medium tomatoes, chopped

6 large eggs

½ cup half and half

½ cup feta cheese, crumbled

¼ cup dill weed

Salt as needed

Ground black pepper as needed

Directions:

Pre-heat your oven to a temperature of 400 degrees Fahrenheit.

Take a large sized ovenproof pan and heat up your olive oil over medium-high heat.

Toss in the onion, garlic, tomatoes and stir fry them for 4 minutes.

While they are being cooked, take a bowl and beat together your eggs, half and half cream and season the mix with some pepper and salt.

Pour the mixture into the pan with your vegetables and top it with crumbled feta cheese and dill weed.

Cover it with the lid and let it cook for 3 minutes.

Place the pan inside your oven and let it bake for 10 minutes .

Serve hot.

Nutrition (Per Serving)

Calories: 191

Fat: 15g

Carbohydrates: 6g

Protein: 9g

Bacon and Brie Omelette Wedges

Difficulty Level: 2/5

Preparation time: 10 minutes

Cooking time: 10 minutes

Servings: 6

Ingredients

2 tablespoons olive oil

7 ounces smoked bacon

6 beaten eggs

Small bunch chives, snipped

3 ½ ounces brie, sliced

1 teaspoon red wine vinegar

1 teaspoon Dijon mustard

1 cucumber, halved, deseeded and sliced diagonally

7 ounces radish, quartered

Directions:

Turn your grill on and set it to high.

Take a small-sized pan and add 1 teaspoon of oil, allow the oil to heat up.

Add lardons and fry until crisp.

Drain the lardon on kitchen paper.

Take another non-sticky cast iron frying pan and place it over grill, heat 2 teaspoons of oil.

Add lardons, eggs, chives, ground pepper to the frying pan.

Cook on LOW until they are semi-set.

Carefully lay brie on top and grill until the Brie sets and is a golden texture .

Remove it from the pan and cut up into wedges.

Take a small bowl and create dressing by mixing olive oil, mustard, vinegar and seasoning.

Add cucumber to the bowl and mix, serve alongside the Omelette wedges.

Enjoy!

Nutrition (Per Serving)

Calories: 35

Fat: 31g

Carbohydrates: 3g

Protein: 25g

Pearl Couscous Salad

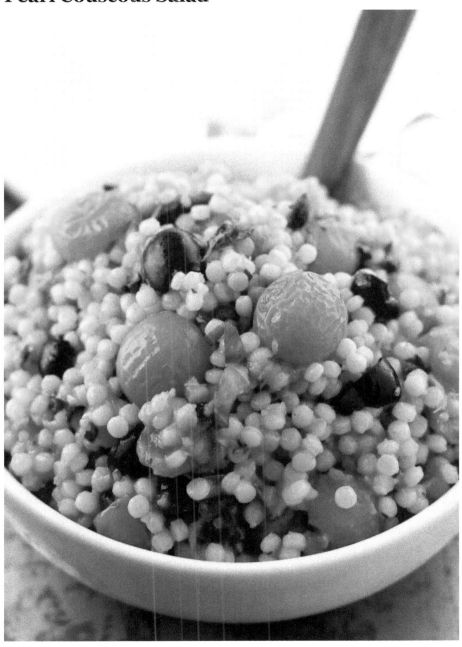

Difficulty Level: 1/5

Preparation time: 15 minutes

Cook Time: 0 minutes

Servings: 6

Ingredients

For Lemon Dill Vinaigrette

Juice of 1 large sized lemon

1/3 cup of extra virgin olive oil

1 teaspoon of dill weed

1 teaspoon of garlic powder

Salt as needed

Pepper

For Israeli Couscous

2 cups of Pearl Couscous

Extra virgin olive oil

2 cups of halved grape tomatoes

Water as needed

1/3 cup of finely chopped red onions

½ of a finely chopped English cucumber

15 ounces of chickpeas

14 ounce can of artichoke hearts (roughly chopped up)

½ cup of pitted Kalamata olives

15-20 pieces of fresh basil leaves, roughly torn and chopped up

3 ounces of fresh baby mozzarella

Directions:

Prepare the vinaigrette by taking a bowl and add the ingredients listed under vinaigrette.

Mix them well and keep aside.

Take a medium-sized heavy pot and place it over medium heat.

Add 2 tablespoons of olive oil and allow it to heat up.

Add couscous and keep cooking until golden brown.

Add 3 cups of boiling water and cook the couscous according to the package instructions.

Once done, drain in a colander and keep aside.

Take another large-sized mixing bowl and add the remaining ingredients except the cheese and basil.

Add the cooked couscous and basil to the mix and mix everything well.

Give the vinaigrette a nice stir and whisk it into the couscous salad.

Mix well.

Adjust the seasoning as required.

Add mozzarella cheese.

Garnish with some basil.

Enjoy!

Nutrition (Per Serving)

Calories: 393

Fat: 13g

Carbohydrates: 57g

Protein: 13g

Simple Coconut Porridge

Difficulty Level: 2/5

Preparation time: 15 minutes

Cooking time: 5

Servings: 6

Ingredients

Powdered erythritol as needed

1 ½ cups almond milk, unsweetened

2 tablespoons vanilla protein powder

3 tablespoons Golden Flaxseed meal

2 tablespoons coconut flour

Directions:

Take a bowl and add flaxseed meal, protein powder, coconut flour and mix well.

Add mix to saucepan (placed over medium heat).

Add almond milk and stir, let the mixture thicken.

Add your desired amount of sweetener and serve.

Enjoy!

Nutrition (Per Serving)

Calories: 259

Fat: 13g

Carbohydrates: 5g

Protein: 16g

Crumbled Feta and Scallions

Difficulty Level: 2/5

Preparation time: 5 minutes

Cooking time: 15 minutes

Servings: 12

Ingredients:

2 tablespoon of unsalted butter (replace with canola oil for full effect)

½ cup of chopped up scallions

1 cup of crumbled feta cheese

8 large sized eggs

2/3 cup of milk

½ teaspoon of dried Italian seasoning

Salt as needed

Freshly ground black pepper as needed

Cooking oil spray

Directions:

Pre-heat your oven to 400 degrees Fahrenheit.

Take a 3-4 ounce muffin pan and grease with cooking oil.

Take a non-stick pan and place it over medium heat.

Add butter and allow the butter to melt.

Add half of the scallions and stir fry.

Keep them to the side.

Take a medium-sized bowl and add eggs, Italian seasoning and milk and whisk well.

Add the stir fried scallions and feta cheese and mix.

Season with pepper and salt .

Pour the mix into the muffin tin.

Transfer the muffin tin to your oven and bake for 15 minutes.

Serve with a sprinkle of scallions.

Enjoy!

Nutrition (Per Serving)

Calories: 106

Fat: 8g

Carbohydrates: 2g

Protein: 7g

Gnocchi Ham Olives

Difficulty Level: 2/5

Preparation time: 5 minutes

Cooking Time: 15 minutes

Servings: 4

Ingredients

2 tablespoons of olive oil

1 medium-sized onion chopped up

3 minced cloves of garlic

1 medium-sized red pepper completely deseeded and finely chopped

1 cup of tomato puree

2 tablespoons of tomato paste

1 pound of gnocchi

1 cup of coarsely chopped turkey ham

½ cup of sliced pitted olives

1 teaspoon of Italian seasoning

Salt as needed

Freshly ground black pepper

Bunch of fresh basil leaves

Directions:

Take a medium-sized sauce pan and place over medium-high heat.

Pour some olive oil and heat it up.

Toss in the bell pepper, onion and garlic and sauté for 2 minutes.

Pour in the tomato puree, gnocchi, tomato paste and add the turkey ham, Italian seasoning and olives.

Simmer the whole mix for 15 minutes, making sure to stir from time to time.

Season the mix with some pepper and salt.

Once done, transfer the mix to a dish and garnish with some basil leaves.

Serve hot and have fun.

Nutrition

Calories: 335

Fat: 12g

Carbohydrates: 45g

Protein: 15g

Spicy Early Morning Seafood Risotto

Difficulty Level: 2/5

Preparation time: 5 minutes

Cooking Time: 15 minutes

Servings: 4

Ingredients

3 cups of clam juice

2 cups of water

2 tablespoons of olive oil

1 medium-sized chopped up onion

2 minced cloves of garlic

1 ½ cups of Arborio Rice

½ cup of dry white wine

1 teaspoon of Saffron

½ teaspoon of ground cumin

½ teaspoon of paprika

1 pound of marinara seafood mix

Salt as needed

Ground pepper as needed

Directions:

Place a saucepan over high heat and pour in your clam juice with water and bring the mixture to a boil.

Remove the heat.

Take a heavy bottomed saucepan and stir fry your garlic and onion in oil over medium heat until a nice fragrance comes off.

Add in the rice and keep stirring for 2-3 minutes until the rice has been fully covered with the oil.

Pour the wine and then add the saffron.

Keep stirring constantly until it is fully absorbed.

Add in the cumin, clam juice, paprika mixture 1 cup at a time, making sure to keep stirring it from time to time.

Cook the rice for 20 minutes until perfect.

Finally, add the seafood marinara mix and cook for another 5-7 minutes.

Season with some pepper and salt.

Transfer the meal to a serving dish.

Serve hot.

Nutrition

Calories: 386

Fat: 7g

Carbohydrates: 55g

Protein: 21g

Rocket Tomatoes and Mushroom Frittata

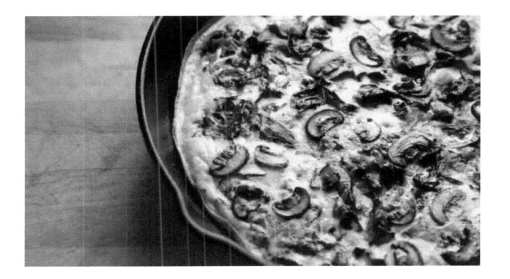

Difficulty Level: 2/5

Preparation time: 5 minutes

Cooking time: 15 minutes

Servings: 4

Ingredients

2 tablespoons of butter (replace with canola oil for full effect)

1 chopped up medium-sized onion

2 minced cloves of garlic

1 cup of coarsely chopped baby rocket tomato

1 cup of sliced button mushrooms

6 large pieces of eggs

½ cup of skim milk

1 teaspoon of dried rosemary

Salt as needed

Ground black pepper as needed

Directions:

Pre-heat your oven to 400 degrees Fahrenheit.

Take a large oven-proof pan and place it over medium-heat.

Heat up some oil.

Stir fry your garlic, onion for about 2 minutes.

Add the mushroom, rosemary and rockets and cook for 3 minutes.

Take a medium-sized bowl and beat your eggs alongside the milk.

Season it with some salt and pepper.

Pour the egg mixture into your pan with the vegetables and sprinkle some Parmesan.

Reduce the heat to low and cover with the lid.

Let it cook for 3 minutes.

Transfer the pan into your oven and bake for 10 minutes until fully settled.

Reduce the heat to low and cover with your lid.

Let it cook for 3 minutes.

Transfer the pan into your oven and then bake for another 10 minutes.

Serve hot.

Nutrition (Per Serving)

Calories: 189

Fat: 13g

Carbohydrates: 6g

Protein: 12g

Yogurt and Cucumber Salad

Difficulty Level: 2/5

Preparation time: 10 minutes

Cooking time: nil

Servings: 4

Ingredients

5-6 small cucumbers, peeled and diced

1 (8 ounces) container plain Greek yogurt

2 garlic cloves, minced

1 tablespoon fresh mint, minced

1 teaspoon dried oregano

Sea salt and fresh black pepper

Directions:

Take a large bowl and add cucumbers, garlic, yogurt, mint, and oregano.

Season with salt and pepper.

Refrigerate the salad for 1 hour and serve.

Enjoy!

Nutrition (Per Serving)

Calories: 74

Fat: 0.7g

Carbohydrates: 16g

Protein: 2g

Breakfast Egg on Avocado

Difficulty Level: 2/5

Preparation Time: 10 minutes

Cooking Time: 15 minutes

Servings: 6

Ingredients:

1 tsp garlic powder

1/2 tsp sea salt

1/4 cup Parmesan cheese (grated or shredded)

1/4 tsp black pepper

3 medium avocados (cut in half, pitted, skin on)

6 medium eggs

Directions:

Prepare muffin tins and preheat the oven to 350oF.

To ensure that the egg would fit inside the cavity of the avocado, lightly scrape off 1/3 of the meat.

Place avocado on muffin tin to ensure that it faces with the top up.

Evenly season each avocado with pepper, salt, and garlic powder.

Add one egg on each avocado cavity and garnish tops with cheese.

Pop in the oven and bake until the egg white is set, about 15 minutes.

Serve and enjoy.

Nutrition:

Calories per serving: 252

Protein: 14.0g

Carbs: 4.0g

Fat: 20.0g

Mediterranean Breakfast Salad

Difficulty Level: 2/5

Preparation Time: 10 minutes

Cooking Time: 20 minutes

Servings: 4

Ingredients:

4 whole eggs

2 cups of cherry tomatoes or heirloom tomatoes cut in half or wedges

10 cups of arugula

A 1/2 chopped seedless cucumber

1 large avocado

1 cup cooked or cooled quinoa

1/2 cup of chopped mixed herbs like dill and mint

1 cup of chopped Almonds

1 lemon

Extra virgin olive oil

Sea salt

Freshly ground black pepper

Directions:

In this recipe, the eggs are the first thing that needs to be cooked. Start with soft boiling the eggs. To do that, you need to get water in a pan and let it sit to boil. Once it starts boiling, reduce the heat to simmer and lower the eggs into the water and let them cook for about 6 minutes. After they are boiled, wash the eggs with cold water and set aside. Peel them when they are cool and ready to use.

Combine quinoa, arugula, cucumbers, and tomatoes in a bowl and add a little bit of olive oil over the top. Toss it with salt and pepper to equally season all of it.

Once all that is done, serve the salad on four plates and garnish it with sliced avocados and the halved eggs. After that, season it with some more pepper and salt.

To top it all off, then use almonds and sprinkle some herbs along with some lemon zest and olive oil.

Nutrition:

Carbohydrate -6.71 g

Protein – 3.4 g

Fat – 3.46 g

Smoked Salmon and Poached Eggs on Toast

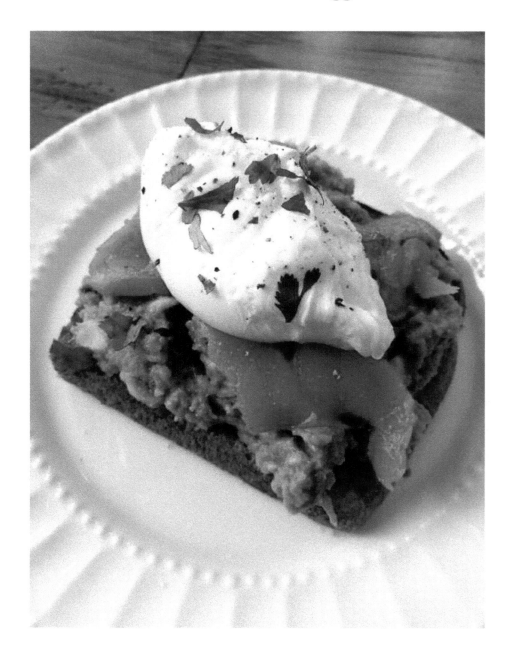

Difficulty Level: 2/5

Preparation Time: 10 minutes

Cooking Time: 4 minutes

Preparation time: 10 minutes

Ingredients:

2 oz avocado smashed

2 slices of bread toasted

Pinch of kosher salt and cracked black pepper

1/4 tsp freshly squeezed lemon juice

2 eggs see notes, poached

3.5 oz smoked salmon

1 TBSP. thinly sliced scallions

Splash of Kikkoman soy sauce optional

Microgreens are optional

Directions:

Take a small bowl and then smash the avocado into it. Then, add the lemon juice and also a pinch of salt into the mixture. Then, mix it well and set aside.

After that, poach the eggs and toast the bread for some time.

Once the bread is toasted, you will have to spread the avocado on both slices and after that, add the smoked salmon to each slice.

Thereafter, carefully transfer the poached eggs to the respective toasts.

Add a splash of Kikkoman soy sauce and some cracked pepper; then, just garnish with scallions and micro greens.

Nutrition:

Carbohydrate – 33.2 g

Protein - 31.1 g

Fat - 21.9 g

Calories: 459.4 kcal

Honey Almond Ricotta Spread with Peaches
Difficulty Level: 2/5

Preparation Time: 5 minutes

Cooking Time: 8 minutes

Preparation time: 5 minutes

Ingredients:

1/2 cup Fisher Sliced Almonds

1 cup whole milk ricotta

1/4 teaspoon almond extract

Zest from an orange, optional

1 teaspoon honey

Hearty whole grain toast

English muffin or bagel

Extra Fisher sliced almonds

Sliced peaches

Extra honey for drizzling

Directions:

Cut peaches into a proper shape and then brush them with olive oil. After that, set it aside.

Take a bowl; combine the ingredients for the filling. Set aside.

Then just pre-heat grill to medium.

Place peaches cut side down onto the greased grill.

Close lid cover and then just grill until the peaches have softened, approximately 6-10 minutes, depending on the size of the peaches.

Then you will have to place peach halves onto a serving plate.

Put a spoon of about 1 tablespoon of ricotta mixture into the cavity (you are also allowed to use a small scooper).

Sprinkle it with slivered almonds, crushed amaretti cookies, and honey. Decorate with the mint leaves.

Nutrition:

Carbohydrate – 19g

Protein - 7g

Fat - 9g

Calories: 187kcal

Mediterranean Eggs Cups

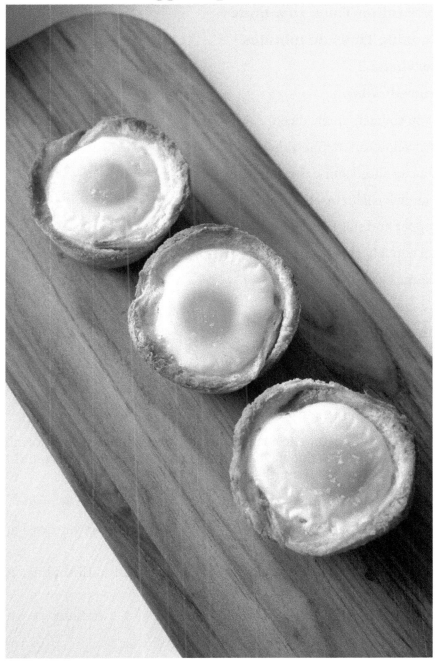

Difficulty Level: 2/5

Preparation Time: 10 minutes

Cooking Time: 20 minutes

Servings: 8

Ingredients:

1 cup spinach, finely diced

1/2 yellow onion, finely diced

1/2 cup sliced sun-dried tomatoes

4 large basil leaves, finely diced

Pepper and salt to taste

1/3 cup feta cheese crumbles

8 large eggs

1/4 cup milk (any kind)

Directions:

You have to heat the oven to 375°F.

Then, roll the dough sheet into a 12x8-inch rectangle

Then, cut in half lengthwise

After that, you will have to cut each half crosswise into 4 pieces, forming 8 (4x3-inch) pieces dough. Then, press each into the bottom and up sides of the ungreased muffin cup.

Trim dough to keep the dough from touching, if essential. Set aside.

Then, you will have to combine the eggs, salt, pepper in the bowl and beat it with a whisk until well mixed. Set aside.

Melt the butter in 12-inch skillet over medium heat until sizzling; add bell peppers.

You will have to cook it, stirring occasionally, 2-3 minutes or until crisply tender.

After that, add spinach leaves; continue cooking until spinach is wilted. Then just add egg mixture and prosciutto.

Divide the mixture evenly among prepared muffin cups.

Finally, bake it for 14-17 minutes or until crust is golden brown.

Nutrition:

Carbohydrate – 13 g

Protein – 9 g

Fat - 16 g

Calories: 240 kcal

Low-Carb Baked Eggs with Avocado and Feta
Difficulty Level: 2/5

Preparation Time: 10 minutes

Cooking Time: 15 minutes

Servings: 2

Ingredients:

1 avocado

4 eggs

2-3 tbsp. crumbled feta cheese

Nonstick cooking spray

Pepper and salt to taste

Directions:

First, you will have to preheat the oven to 400 degrees F.

After that, when the oven is on the proper temperature, you will have to put the gratin dishes right on the baking sheet.

Then, leave the dishes to heat in the oven for almost 10 minutes

After that process, you need to break the eggs into individual ramekins.

Then, let the avocado and eggs come to room temperature for at least 10 minutes

Then, peel the avocado properly and cut it each half into 6-8 slices

You will have to remove the dishes from the oven and spray them with the non-stick spray

Then, you will have to arrange all the sliced avocados in the dishes and tip two eggs into each dish

Sprinkle with feta, add pepper and salt to taste

Last, bake it for 12-15 minutes or until egg whites are set and the egg yolks are done to your liking. Serve hot.

Nutrition:

Carbohydrate – 9.3g

Protein – 11.3g

Fat – 23.5g

Calories: 280 kcal

Mediterranean Eggs White Breakfast Sandwich with Roasted Tomatoes

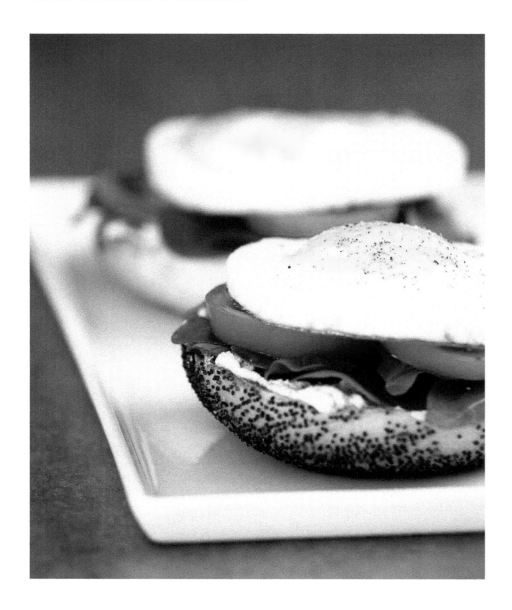

Difficulty Level: 2/5

Preparation Time: 15 minutes

Cooking Time: 10 minutes

Servings: 2

Ingredients:

Salt and pepper to taste

¼ cup egg whites

1 teaspoon chopped fresh herbs like rosemary, basil, parsley,

1 whole grain seeded ciabatta roll

1 teaspoon butter

1-2 slices Muenster cheese

1 tablespoon pesto

About ½ cup roasted tomatoes

10 ounces grape tomatoes

1 tablespoon extra-virgin olive oil

Black pepper and salt to taste

Directions:

First, you will have to melt the butter over medium heat in the small nonstick skillet.

Then, mix the egg whites with pepper and salt.

Then, sprinkle it with the fresh herbs

After that cook it for almost 3-4 minutes or until the eggs are done, then flip it carefully

Meanwhile, toast ciabatta bread in the toaster

After that, you will have to place the egg on the bottom half of the sandwich rolls, then top with cheese

Add roasted tomatoes and the top half of roll.

To make a roasted tomato, preheat the oven to 400 degrees.

Then, slice the tomatoes in half lengthwise.

Place on the baking sheet and drizzle with the olive oil.

Season it with pepper and salt and then roast in the oven for about 20 minutes. Skins will appear wrinkled when done.

Nutrition:

Carbohydrate – 51g

Protein – 21g

Fat – 24g

Calories: 458

Greek Yogurt Pancakes

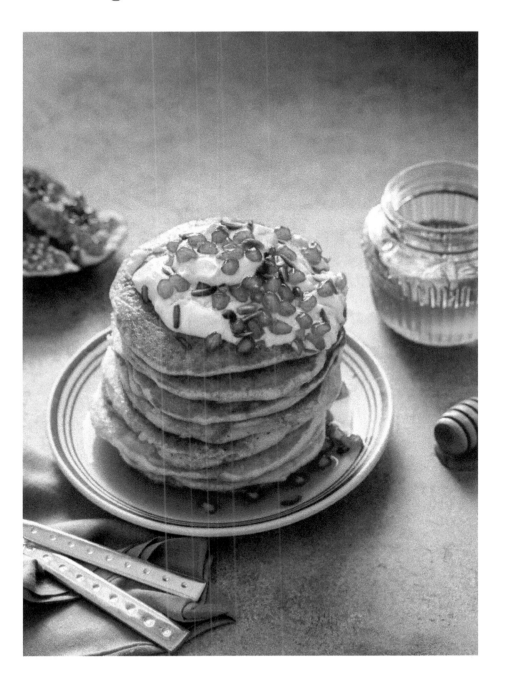

Difficulty Level: 2/5

Preparation Time: 10 minutes

Cooking Time: 5 minutes

Servings: 2

Ingredients:

1 cup all-purpose flour

1 cup whole-wheat flour

1/4 teaspoon salt

4 teaspoons baking powder

1 Tablespoon sugar

1 1/2 cups unsweetened almond milk

2 teaspoons vanilla extract

2 large eggs

1/2 cup plain 2% Greek yogurt

Fruit, for serving

Maple syrup, for serving

Directions:

First, you will have to pour the curds into the bowl and mix them well until creamy.

After that, you will have to add egg whites and mix them well until combined.

Then take a separate bowl, pour the wet mixture into the dry mixture. Stir to combine. The batter will be extremely thick.

Then, simply spoon the batter onto the sprayed pan heated to medium-high.

The batter must make 4 large pancakes.

Then, you will have to flip the pancakes once when they start to bubble a bit on the surface. Cook until golden brown on both sides.

Nutrition:

Carbohydrate – 52g

Protein – 14g

Fat – 5g

Calories: 165.7

Mediterranean Feta and Quinoa Egg Muffins

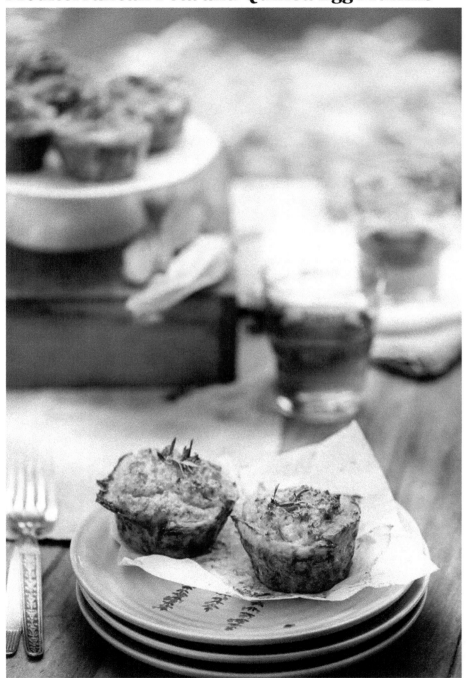

Difficulty Level: 2/5

Preparation Time: 15 minutes

Cooking Time: 15 minutes

Servings: 12

Ingredients:

2 cups baby spinach finely chopped

1 cup chopped or sliced cherry tomatoes

1/2 cup finely chopped onion

1 tablespoon chopped fresh oregano

1 cup crumbled feta cheese

1/2 cup chopped \'7bpitted\'7d kalamata olives

2 teaspoons high oleic sunflower oil

1 cup cooked quinoa

8 eggs

1/4 teaspoon salt

Directions:

Pre-heat oven to 350 degrees Fahrenheit, and then prepare 12 silicone muffin holders on the baking sheet, or just grease a 12-cup muffin tin with oil and set aside.

Finely chop the vegetables and then heat the skillet to medium.

After that, add the vegetable oil and onions and sauté for 2 minutes.

Then, add tomatoes and sauté for another minute, then add spinach and sauté until wilted, about 1 minute.

Place the beaten egg into a bowl and then add lots of vegetables like feta cheese, quinoa, veggie mixture as well as salt, and then stir well until everything is properly combined.

Pour the ready mixture into greased muffin tins or silicone cups, dividing the mixture equally. Then, bake it in an oven for 30 minutes or so, or until the eggs set nicely, and the muffins turn a light golden brown in color.

Nutrition:

Carbohydrate – 5g

Protein – 6g

Fat – 7g

Calories: 113kcal

Pastry-Less Spanakopita

Difficulty Level: 2/5

Preparation Time: 5 minutes

Cooking Time: 20 minutes

Servings: 4

Ingredients:

1/8 teaspoons black pepper, add as per taste

1/3 cup of Extra virgin olive oil

4 lightly beaten eggs

7 cups of Lettuce, preferably a spring mix (mesclun)

1/2 cup of crumbled Feta cheese

1/8 teaspoon of Sea salt, add to taste

1 finely chopped medium Yellow onion

Directions:

For this delicious recipe, you need to first start by preheating the oven to 180C and grease the flan dish.

Once done, pour the extra virgin olive oil into a large saucepan and heat it over medium heat with the onions, until they are translucent. To that, add greens and keep stirring until all the ingredients are wilted.

After completing that, you should season it with salt and pepper and transfer the greens to the prepared dish and sprinkle on some feta cheese.

Pour the eggs and bake it for 20 minutes till it is cooked through and slightly brown.

Nutrition:

Carbohydrate -7.3 g

Protein – 11.2 g

Fat – 27.9 g

Calories: 325

Coconut Risotto

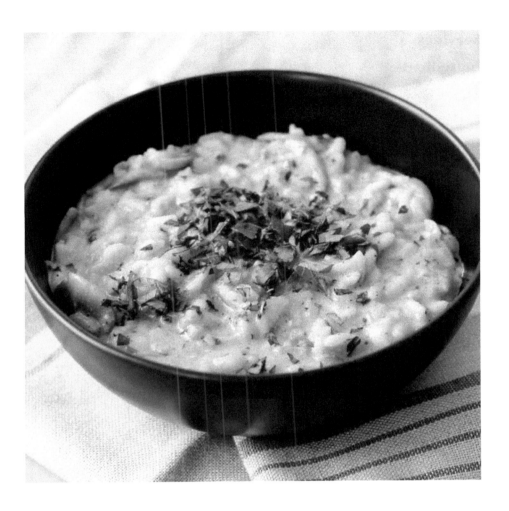

Difficulty Level: 2/5

Preparation time: 5 Minutes

Cooking time: 5 Minutes

Servings: 4

Ingredients:

2 Cups Coconut Milk

½ Cup Arborio Rice

2 Tablespoons Coconut Sugar

1 Teaspoon Vanilla Extract

¼ Cup Coconut Flakes, Toasted for Garnish

Directions:

Throw all of your ingredients into the Pressure Pot and then cook on high pressure for five minutes.

Allow for a natural pressure release for twenty minutes before serving with coconut flakes.

Nutrition:

Calories: 532,

Protein: 5.9 Grams,

Fat: 40.4 Grams,

Carbs: 42.1 Grams,

Sodium: 25 mg

Breakfast Quinoa

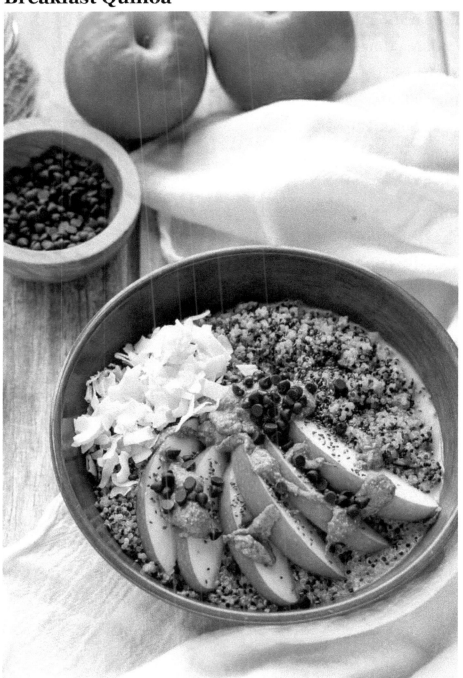

Difficulty Level: 2/5

Preparation time: 5 Minutes

Cooking time: 10 Minutes

Servings: 4

Ingredients:

1 Cup Quinoa, Rinsed & Drained

3 Cups Almond Milk, Vanilla

¼ Cup Almonds

1 Cup Blackberries, Chopped

¼ Teaspoon Cinnamon

Directions:

Start by placing your quinoa in your Pressure Pot, and then pour in your milk. Add in your cinnamon. Seal your Pressure Pot before setting it to manual settings.

Cook at high pressure for two minutes before allowing for a natural pressure release.

Top with almonds and berries before serving.

Nutrition:

Calories: 267,

Protein: 8.5 Grams,

Fat: 7.6 Grams,

Carbs: 35 Grams,

Sodium: 140 Grams

Western Omelette

Difficulty Level: 2/5

Preparation time: 5 Minutes

Cooking time: 20 Minutes

Servings: 4

Ingredients:

1 green pepper

5 eggs

½ yellow onion, diced

3-ounces Parmesan cheese, shredded

1 teaspoon butter

1 teaspoon oregano, dried

1 teaspoon cilantro, dried

1 teaspoon olive oil

3 tablespoons cream cheese

Directions:

In a bowl, add the eggs and whisk them. Sprinkle the cilantro, oregano, and cream cheese into the eggs. Add the shredded parmesan and mix the egg mixture well.

Preheat your air fryer to 360°Fahrenheit. Pour the egg mixture into the air fryer basket tray and place it into the air fryer. Cook the omelet for 10-minutes.

Meanwhile, chop the green pepper and dice the onion. Pour olive oil into a skillet and preheat well over medium heat. Add the chopped green pepper and onion to skillet and roast for 8-minutes. Stir veggies often.

Remove the omelet from air fryer basket tray and place it on a serving plate. Add the roasted vegetables and serve warm.

Nutrition:

Calories: 204,

Total Fat: 14.9g,

Carbs: 4.3g,

Protein: 14.8g

Breakfast Coconut Porridge

Difficulty Level: 2/5

Preparation time: 5 Minutes

Cooking time: 10 Minutes

Servings: 4

Ingredients:

1 cup coconut milk

3 tablespoons blackberries

2 tablespoons walnuts

1 teaspoon butter

1 teaspoon ground cinnamon

5 tablespoons chia seeds

3 tablespoons coconut flakes

¼ teaspoon salt

Directions:

Pour the coconut milk into the air fryer basket tray. Add the coconut, salt, chia seeds, ground cinnamon, and butter. Ground up the walnuts and add them to the air fryer basket tray. Sprinkle the mixture with salt.

Mash the blackberries with a fork and add them also to the air fryer basket tray. Cook the porridge at 375°Fahrenheit for 7-minutes. When the cook time is over, remove the air fryer basket from air fryer and allow to sit and rest for 5-minutes. Stir porridge with a wooden spoon and serve warm.

Nutrition:

Calories: 169,

Total Fat: 18.2g,

Carbs: 9.3g,

Protein: 4.2g

Egg Butter

Difficulty Level: 2/5

Preparation time: 5 Minutes

Cooking time: 20 Minutes

Servings: 4

Ingredients:

4 eggs

4 tablespoons butter

1 teaspoon salt

Directions:

Cover the air fryer basket with foil and place the eggs there. Transfer the air fryer basket into the air fryer and cook the eggs for 17 minutes at 320°Fahrenheit. When the time is over, remove the eggs from the air fryer basket and put them in cold water to chill them. After this, peel the eggs and chop them up finely. Combine the chopped eggs with butter and add salt. Mix it until you get the spread texture. Serve the egg butter with the keto almond bread.

Nutrition:

Calories: 164,

Total Fat: 8.5g,

Carbs: 2.67g,

Protein: 3g

Flax Meal Porridge

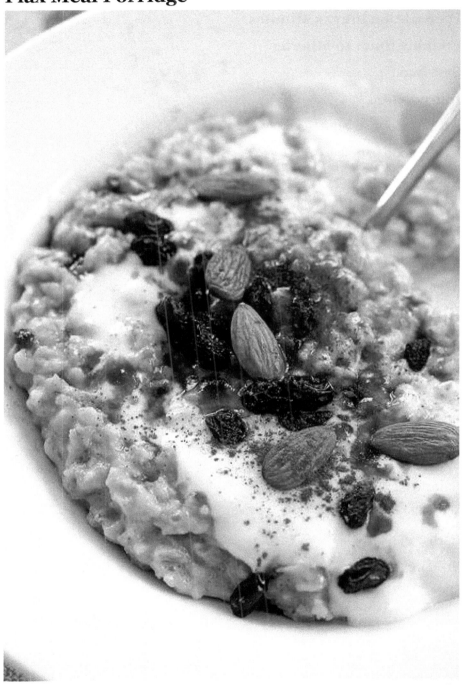

Difficulty Level: 2/5

Preparation time: 5 Minutes

Cooking time: 10 Minutes

Servings: 4

Ingredients:

2 tablespoons sesame seeds

½ teaspoon vanilla extract

1 tablespoon butter

1 tablespoon liquid Stevia

3 tablespoons flax meal

1 cup almond milk

4 tablespoons chia seeds

Directions:

Preheat your air fryer to 375°Fahrenheit. Put the sesame seeds, chia seeds, almond milk, flax meal, liquid Stevia and butter into the air fryer basket tray.

Add the vanilla extract and cook porridge for 8-minutes. When porridge is cooked stir it carefully then allow it to rest for 5-minutes before serving.

Nutrition:

Calories: 298,

Total Fat: 26.7g,

Carbs: 13.3 g,

Protein: 6.2g

Scrambled Pancake Hash

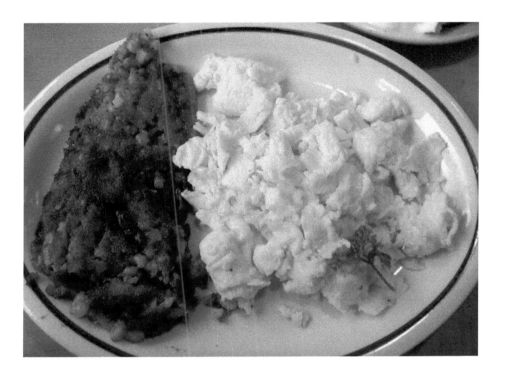

Difficulty Level: 2/5

Preparation time: 5 Minutes

Cooking time: 10 Minutes

Servings: 4

Ingredients:

1 egg

¼ cup heavy cream

5 tablespoons butter

1 cup coconut flour

1 teaspoon ground ginger

1 teaspoon salt

1 tablespoon apple cider vinegar

1 teaspoon baking soda

Directions:

Combine the salt, baking soda, ground ginger and flour in a mixing bowl. In a separate bowl crack, the egg into it. Add butter and heavy cream. Mix well using a hand mixer. Combine the liquid and dry mixtures and stir until smooth.

Preheat your air fryer to 400°Fahrenheit. Pour the pancake mixture into the air fryer basket tray. Cook the pancake hash for 4-minutes. After this, scramble the pancake hash well and continue to cook for another 5-minutes more. When dish is cooked, transfer it to serving plates, and serve hot!

Nutrition:

Calories: 178,

Total Fat: 13.3g,

Carbohydrates: 10.7g,

Protein: 4.4g

Zucchini and Quinoa Pan

Difficulty Level: 2/5

Preparation time: 10 minutes

Cooking time: 20 minutes

Servings: 4

Ingredients:

1 tablespoon olive oil

2 garlic cloves, minced

1 cup quinoa

1 zucchini, roughly cubed

2 tablespoons basil, chopped

¼ cup green olives, pitted and chopped

1 tomato, cubed

½ cup feta cheese, crumbled

2 cups water

1 cup canned garbanzo beans, drained and rinsed

A pinch of salt and black pepper

Directions:

Heat up a pan with the oil over medium-high heat, add the garlic and quinoa and brown for 3 minutes.

Add the water, zucchinis, salt and pepper, toss, bring to a simmer and cook for 15 minutes.

Add the rest of the ingredients, toss, divide everything between plates and serve for breakfast.

Nutrition:

Calories 310,

Fat 11,

Fiber 6,

Carbs 42,

Protein 11

Banana-Coconut Breakfast

Difficulty Level: 2/5

Preparation time: 5 Minutes

Cooking time: 20 Minutes

Servings: 4

Ingredients:

1 ripe banana

1 cup desiccated coconut

1 cup coconut milk

3 tablespoons raisins, chopped

2 tablespoon ground flax seed

1 teaspoon vanilla

A dash of cinnamon

A dash of nutmeg

Salt to taste

Directions:

Place all ingredients in a deep pan.

Allow to simmer for 3 minutes on low heat.

Place in individual containers.

Put a label and store in the fridge.

Allow to thaw at room temperature before heating in the microwave oven.

Nutrition:

Calories per serving:279;

Carbs: 25.46g;

Protein: 6.4g;

Fat: g;

Fiber: 5.9g

Morning Time Sausages

Difficulty Level: 2/5

Preparation time: 5 Minutes

Cooking time: 15 Minutes

Servings: 4

Ingredients:

7ounces ground chicken

7ounces ground pork

1 teaspoon ground coriander

1 teaspoon basil, dried

½ teaspoon nutmeg

1 teaspoon olive oil

1 teaspoon minced garlic

1 tablespoon coconut flour

1 egg

1 teaspoon soy sauce

1 teaspoon sea salt

½ teaspoon ground black pepper

Directions:

Combine the ground pork, chicken, soy sauce, ground black pepper, garlic, basil, coriander, nutmeg, sea salt, and egg. Add the coconut flour and mix the mixture well to combine. Preheat your air fryer to 360°Fahrenheit. Make medium-sized sausages with the ground meat mixture. Spray the inside of the air fryer basket tray with the olive oil. Place prepared sausages into the air fryer basket and place inside of air fryer. Cook the sausages for 6-minutes. Turn the sausages over and cook for 6-minutes more. When the cook time is completed, let the sausages chill for a little bit. Serve warm.

Nutrition:

Calories: 156,

Total Fat: 7.5g,

Carbs: 1.3g,

Protein: 20.2g

Baked Bacon Egg Cups

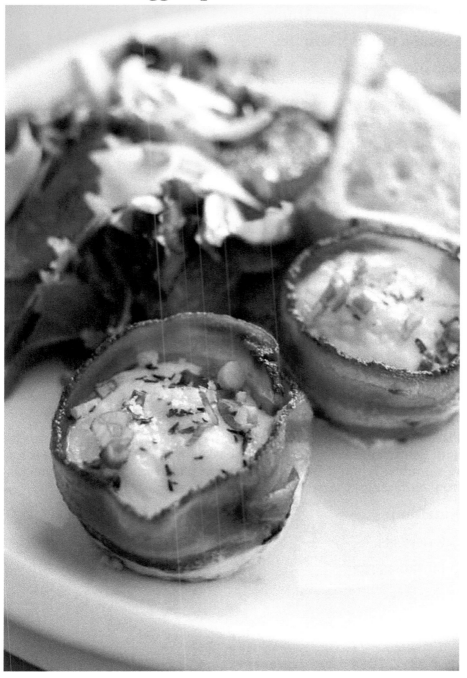

Difficulty Level: 2/5

Preparation time: 5 Minutes

Cooking time: 15 Minutes

Servings: 4

Ingredients:

2 eggs

1 tablespoon chives, fresh, chopped

½ teaspoon paprika

½ teaspoon cayenne pepper

3-ounces cheddar cheese, shredded

½ teaspoon butter

¼ teaspoon salt

4-ounces bacon, cut into tiny pieces

Directions:

Slice bacon into tiny pieces and sprinkle it with cayenne pepper, salt, and paprika. Mix the chopped bacon. Spread butter in bottom of ramekin dishes and beat the eggs there. Add the chives and shredded cheese. Add the chopped bacon over egg mixture in ramekin dishes.

Place the ramekins in your air fryer basket. Preheat your air fryer to 360°Fahrenheit. Place the air fryer basket in your air fryer and cook for 12-minutes. When the cook time is completed, remove the ramekins from air fryer and serve warm.

Nutrition:

Calories: 553,

Total Fat: 43.3g,

Carbs: 2.3g,

Protein: 37.3g

Coconut Yogurt

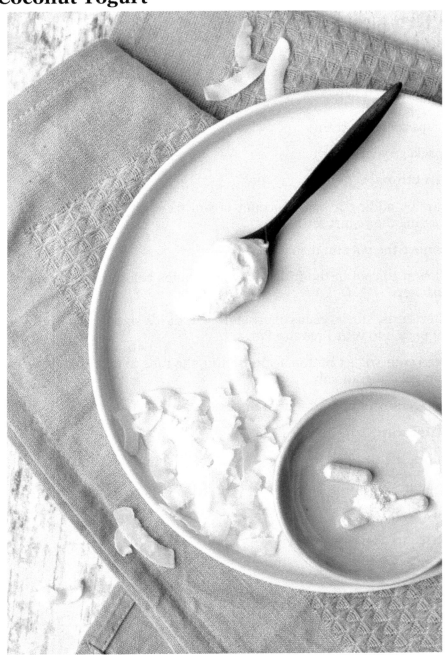

Difficulty Level: 2/5

Preparation time: 5 Minutes

Cooking time: 30 Minutes

Servings: 4

Ingredients:

1 tablespoon gelatin

3 cups coconut cream

1 package yogurt starter

Directions:

Start by adding in your coconut cream to your Pressure Pot before pressing the yogurt setting.

Remove the pot and turn it off.

Allow it to cool in the fridge for ten minutes before moving onto the next step.

Afterwards, stir in your yogurt starter until it's smooth, and put your pot back into your Pressure Pot.

Press your yogurt button again, setting the time to eight hours. Stir in your gelatin gradually.

Refrigerate for at least four hours before serving.

Nutrition:

Calories: 421,

Protein: 5.6 Grams,

Fat: 42.9 Grams,

Carbs: 10.2 Grams,

Sodium: 32 mg

Squash & Apple Porridge

Difficulty Level: 2/5

Preparation time: 5 Minutes

Cooking time: 10 Minutes

Servings: 4

Ingredients:

1 Delicate Squash, Peeled

4 Apples, Cored & Sliced

1/8 Teaspoon Ground Ginger

½ Teaspoon Cinnamon

2 Tablespoons Maple Syrup

Directions:

Start by placing your apples and squash in your Pressure Pot before adding in a cup of water.

Sprinkle with ginger, a dash of salt and cinnamon before sealing your pot and setting it to manual. Cook on high pressure for eight minutes.

Allow for a natural pressure release and then slice the squash.

Transfer your squash and everything else in a blender, pulsing until smooth.

Drizzle with maple syrup before serving.

Nutrition:

Calories: 151,

Protein: 1.2 Grams,

Fat: 0.5 Grams,

Carbs: 39.4 Grams,

Sodium: 48 mg

Mesmerizing Brussels and Pistachios

Difficulty Level: 2/5

Preparation time: 5 Minutes

Cooking time: 20 Minutes

Servings: 4

Ingredients

1 pound Brussels sprouts, tough bottom trimmed and halved lengthwise

1 tablespoon extra-virgin olive oil

Salt and pepper as needed

½ cup roasted pistachios, chopped

Juice of ½ lemon

Directions:

Preheat your oven to 400 degrees Fahrenheit

Line a baking sheet with aluminum foil and keep it on the side

Take a large bowl and add Brussels sprouts with olive oil and coat well

Season sea salt, pepper, spread veggies evenly on sheet

Bake for 15 minutes until lightly caramelized

Remove oven and transfer to a serving bowl

Toss with pistachios and lemon juice

Serve warm and enjoy!

Nutrition:

Calories: 126 ,

Fat: 7g,

Carbohydrates: 14g

Chicken & Quinoa Stew

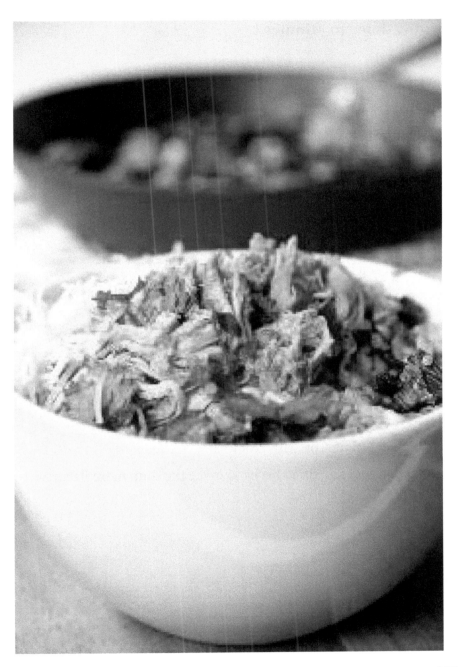

Difficulty Level: 2/5

Preparation time: 5 Minutes

Cooking time: 30 Minutes

Servings: 4

Ingredients:

1 1/4 lb. chicken thigh fillet, sliced into strips

4 cups butternut squash, chopped

4 cups chicken stock

1 cup onion, chopped

½ cup uncooked quinoa

Directions:

Put the chicken in the Pressure Pot.

Add the rest of the ingredients except the quinoa.

Cover the pot. Turn it to manual and cook at high pressure for 8 minutes.

Release the pressure naturally.

Stir the quinoa into the stew.

Set it to sauté and Cook for 15 minutes. Serve and enjoy

Serving Suggestion: Top with croutons.

Tip: Add bay leaf and dried herbs to make the soup more flavorful.

Nutrition:

Calories 251 ,

Total Fat 4.2g ,

Saturated Fat 1g ,

Cholesterol 73mg ,

Sodium 574mg ,

Total Carbohydrate 22.3g ,

Dietary Fiber 3.3g ,

Total Sugars 3.3g ,

Protein 31g ,

Potassium 623mg

Lightning Source UK Ltd.
Milton Keynes UK
UKHW020749030621
384855UK00001B/91